D1765222

The Ultimate Low Carb Cookbook

Delicious and Healthy Low Carb Recipes
incl. 30 Days Low Carb Diet Challenge

1st Edition

Sarah Amber Patterson

Copyright © [2018] [Sarah Amber Patterson]

All rights reserved

All rights for this book here presented belong exclusively to the author.
Usage or reproduction of the text is forbidden and requires a clear consent of
the author in case of expectations.

ISBN- 9781091521537

Table of contents

Introduction...1

What is Low Carb?...1

Carbs – What do you need to know?..2

What happens in our body?...3

Is Low Carb really healthy?...4

    Nervous System Function:..4

    Cholesterol level:...4

    Ketosis:...5

    Digestion:...5

What am I allowed to eat? 7

Meat...7

Fish and seafood 8

Vegetables 8

Fruits 8

What to keep ones hands off 8

How many Carbs per Day? 11

How to start with Low Carb? 13

Recipes for Breakfast 15

One Minute Muffin 16

Western-Style Breakfast Burritos 17

Avocado Harissa Toasts with Poached Egg 19

Six ingredient sausage potato pie 20

Jelly 'n Peanut Butter Chia Pudding 22

Recipes for Lunch 25

Grilled Chicken with Spinach and Melted Mozzarella 26

Eggocado 28

Portabella Mini Pizzas 29

Venetian Shrimp and Scallops 31

Moroccan Meatballs 33

Recipes for Dinner.. 35

Cheese and Pepper (Cacio e Pepe) Spaghetti Squash 36

One-pan cinnamon chipotle baked pork chops 37

Oven Roasted Cauliflower with Garlic, Olive Oil and Lemon Juice 39

Spinach Souffle as easy as Pie 41

Spicy Garlic Shrimp in under 5 minutes 42

Recipes for Desserts.. 43

Low Carb trifle...44

Chocolate Mousse...45

Banana Waffle..47

Recipes for Snacks.. 49

Spicy almond and seed mix.. 50

Garlic Bread 51

Recipes for Smoothies 53

Peppermint Pattie Smoothie... 54

Choc Peanut Butter Smoothie... 55

30 Day Meal Plan **57**

DAY 1 59

DAY 2 60

DAY 3 62

DAY 4 64

DAY 5 65

DAY 6 66

DAY 7 68

DAY 8 69

DAY 9 71

DAY 10 73

DAY 11 74

DAY 12 75

DAY 13 76

DAY 14 77

DAY 15 78

DAY 16 79

DAY 17 80

DAY 18 81

DAY 19 82

DAY 20 83

DAY 21 84

DAY 22 85

DAY 23 87

DAY 24 88

DAY 25 90

DAY 26 92

DAY 27 93

DAY 28 94

DAY 29 95

DAY 30 96

Disclaimer **97**

Imprint **99**

Introduction

You've decided to check out the carbohydrate debacle that's been impacting what seems to be everyone's daily eating of late. But what is it really all about? We'll endeavour to explain this interesting way of fuelling your body (without packing on the fat) in a condensed and easily understood manner.

What is Low Carb?

Low-carb quite simply restricts carbohydrates in the diet and encourages real food, rich in protein, fat, and healthy vegetables. Not all carbohydrates should be avoided entirely though, but definitely those found in bread, pasta, and sugary foods. You won't battle to find a low-carb diet, of which there are many and varied options. Low Carb is a healthy way of eating, that calls for moderation and wise choices.

Carbs – What do you need to know?

The bod's primary source of energy comes in the form of carbohydrates. These include both **simple sugars** and the larger **complex carbohydrates**. The body may convert carbohydrates into glycogen, which is stored for later use, or it may use the carbs immediately. When you take in too many carbohydrates for the body to use immediately or to store as glycogen, it is converted to fat.

Simple sugars are made up of one or two sugar units, glucose being a simple monosaccharide (single-sugar). The body and brain use simple sugar for daily energy. Simple sugars are easily digestible into glucose and fructose, are water-soluble and quickly absorbed into the bloodstream. Single sugars (monosaccharides) include fructose (fruit and veg), galactose (milk), and ribose (RNA in the body's cells). These single sugars can combine to form two-sugars (disaccharides) such as **lactose** (milk sugar) = glucose + galactose; **sucrose** (table sugar) = glucose + fructose; **maltose** (malt sugar) = malted cereals.

When long chains of single sugar units are built up, these become **complex carbohydrates**. These chains can also form branches. Complex carbohydrates include **starch** (potatoes, rice, wheat, carrots, and corn) which are found in plants and are made up of many glucose units linked together. These are not water-soluble; **glycogen**, glucose stored as energy and found in the muscle and liver of animals; **cellulose** is basically the plant skeleton and keeps plants in shape. Cellulose is not digestible but is a principal in dietary fibre.

What happens in our body?

When understanding how the body metabolises whatever we eat, it is important to remember that we have evolved from a species who were never assured of where their next meal would be coming from.

The moment food is placed in the mouth, every bit of it is broken down to be used by the body. Along the metabolic route, proteins, carbohydrates, and fats all play a unique role as nutrients. In a diet where all three nutrients are sufficient, proteins become the raw materials used for essential biological equipment, hormones and muscle, while fats and carbohydrates become the source of energy. All not being equal however, proteins will provide energy in the event of the body does not have enough carbohydrates or fats. The human body has the ability to effectively store fats. Conversely, the body has a limited capacity to store carbohydrates, which is the reason they are so readily used for energy. Carbs are always burned first to fuel the body. Only when carbs are insufficient does the body turn to using fat and proteins as fuel.o.o.o.

After digestion, carbs are converted into glucose which makes quick stop in the liver after entering the human circulatory system. This is the point at which carbs affect blood sugar levels. Whatever glucose is left over after the liver stores excess to maintain blood sugar levels between meals is stored as fat for future needs. Nothing is wasted when it comes to carbs. In the absence of carbs, fat fuels the body, and when that is scarce, fat tissue is broken down for energy. Certain cells, like the brain cells, can however not function on fatty acids, and need glucose. When carbs are low, these cells need the body to produce ketone bodies which are fat like molecules that can produce the energy needed by those body parts that cannot metabolize fatty acids.

Is Low Carb really healthy?

As with anything when it comes to nourishing the body, moderation is key. Of course, insufficient carb intake will impact your health negatively and may affect the kidneys, brain, and heart. Being a main source of energy, it is also the chief supplier of the body's calories. Inadequate carb intake will lead to extreme fatigue and loss of focus, which will negatively affect digestion, too, because of fibre deficiency.

Other points of concern could be:

Nervous System Function:

carbohydrates fuel the neurons to run the nervous system. Too few carbs will result in tiredness, lack of concentration and impaired motor skills.

Cholesterol level:

low-carb usually equates to abnormally high fat intake from animal sources. While these are carb-free, they do contain saturated fat and natural trans-fat. Saturated and trans fats raise cholesterol levels, while trans fats also lower high-density lipoprotein, the "good cholesterol" that protects the heart.

Ketosis:

A natural by-product of fat metabolism is ketone. The body depends on ketones for a limited time, and when ketones build up in the blood, the body goes into a state of ketosis. This typically occurs with a carb intake of less than 20 grams a day, and manifests in headaches, nausea, fatigue and possible kidney damage over prolonged periods.

Digestion:

Fibre is one of those carbs that does not convert to glucose. Only plant-based foods, such as fresh produce, beans and lentils, contain fibre, but they are also high in carbohydrates. It follows then that low card diets may be fibre-deficient, resulting in constipation or diarrhoea. Prolonged deficiency could cause diverticular disease, with food sticking in the in-testinal tract. 14 grams of fibre per 1,000 calories is necessary in a healthy diet.

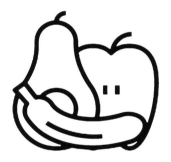

What am I allowed to eat?

In a nutshell (pun intended), these are suggested to include in any healthy low-carb diet:

Meat

Beef is carb-free. Grass-fed and grass-finished beef is best but may be unaffordable for some to maintain. Most pork products are carb-free or very low in carb grams, including bacon, which is however high in sodium. Game meats (venison, antelope, moose, rabbit) are high in protein and carbohydrate-free.

Poultry meat or eggs, including chicken, duck, turkey, goose, ostrich and pheasant, are naturally carb-free. Cooking methods do however add carbs: 85 grams of roasted chicken is carb-free while fried pushes it to 8 grams of carbs.

Fish and seafood

Seafood is king! Fish and shellfish are all high in protein, either low-fat or packed with omega 3 fatty acids, and almost carb-free.

Vegetables

The accepted rule is that if the vegetable grows above ground (spinach), it's good for low-carb eating. Not lettuce, though. Veggies grown below ground (carrots) are generally best not included.

Fruits

Fruits are like nature's candy. The carbs in fruit are mostly sugars. Berries are good in moderation as fruits go. Depending on how many carbs your diet allows, you may be allowed up to 3 portions a day. Raspberries are the best option for low carb, and bananas are of the highest in carbs.

What to keep ones hands off

Some foods on this list may be allowed, depending on your carb allowance per day. Generally speaking these should be limited or avoided altogether:

- Breads and grains
- Pasta
- Cereal
- Certain fruits

- Starchy vegetables

- Beer

- Sweetened yoghurt

- Juice

- Low fat or fat free salad dressings

- Beans and legumes

- Honey and any form of sugar

- Chips and Crackers

- Milk

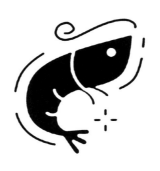

How many Carbs per Day?

Since body type, gender, size and activity levels all impact calorie requirements, there is no hard and fast rule as to how many carbs you, as a unique individual, should endeavour to stick to. Between 45 and 65% of calories should be from carbohydrates. Carbs contain 4 calories/gram, except fibre which is calorie-free. A 2,000-calorie diet therefore equates to 225 - 325 grams of carbohydrates (900 - 1,300 calories). Whole foods are your best option for carbs, so stick to fresh fruit, vegetables, grains and legumes, which offer healthy amounts of carbohydrates, fibre, minerals and essential vitamins.

How to start with Low Carb?

A diet restricted in sugar and starches stabilizes blood sugar and leads to a drop in the fat-storing hormone, insulin. Fat burning increases and satiation is increased which means food intake should decrease and lead to weight loss.

Blood sugar is a tricky variable. As such, while it is safe for most to embark on a low-carb diet, some situations may require preparation or adaptation:

- While medicated for diabetes or high blood pressure;
- While breastfeeding.

You will probably have heard about various low carb diets out there. If you haven't been sold on any specific one, it would be best to kick off with a standard low carb diet that allows for up to 100 grams of carbs daily. Jumping in the deep end with a very limited carb intake has the following bad side:

- **Low Carb Flu** will leave you feeling like giving up. Press on, it only lasts a short time. You can expect fatigue, headaches, nausea, irritability and possibly a cough;
- **Yeast-death:** carbs breed yeast, and these will likely die off if you drastically decrease carb intake. It won't be a pleasant experience but will also be short lived.

The good news is that our meal plan will be more of a dipping your toe in than launching you into the deep end. That being said, we would suggest some easing in. Easing in ultimately depends on your goals as well as your personality but bear in mind regardless that general health should be your ultimate goal. Ditch any foods with added sugar, bread, beer, and pasta.

RECIPES FOR BREAKFAST

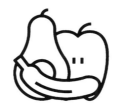

One Minute Muffin

Time: 15 minutes | Serves 4

Net carbs: 2% (5g), Fibre: 12% (3g), Fat: 9% (6g), Protein: 14% (7g), Kcal: 54

Ingredients:

♦ 4 eggs

♦ 8 tsp coconut flour

♦ pinch baking soda

♦ pinch salt

Preparation:

1. Lightly grease a ramekin dish with butter/coconut oil and preheat oven to 400°F (200°C) unless microwaving.

2. Mix all the ingredients with a fork in a mug until free of lumps.

3. Pour mixture into the greased ramekin and bake at 400°F (200°C) for 12 mins, or microwave for 1 min on high.

Western-Style Breakfast Burritos

Time: 15 minutes | Serves 4

Net carbs: 8% (25.3 g), Fibre: 12% (2.9g), Fat: 14% (8.9g), Protein: 31% (15.7g), Kcal: 220

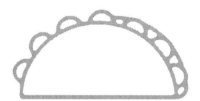

Ingredients:

♦ 1 yellow onion

♦ ½ bell pepper, green variety

♦ 60g low-sodium lean ham

♦ 4 large eggs

♦ 2 tsps. unsalted butter

♦ ½ cup cheddar cheese, low-fat

♦ black pepper to taste

♦ 4 mini wheat tortillas

♦ ¼ cup salsa

Preparation:

1. Finely chop the onion, bell pepper, and ham. Set aside.

2. Whisk the 4 eggs and add the chopped ham, onion, and bell pepper.

3. Place a non-stick skillet over low to medium heat and heat the. Add the eggs and veggie mixture. Cook for 1 ½ to 2 minutes until the eggs are done.

4. Sprinkle with cheese and sprinkle on black pepper to taste.

5. Place equal measures of egg mixture down the centre of each tortilla and top with 1 tbsp salsa. Roll tortilla burrito style. Serve with berries or other fresh fruit as desired.

Avocado Harissa Toasts with Poached Egg

Time: 10 minutes | Serves 4

Net carbs: 19g, Fibre: 5g, Fat: 17g, Protein: 14g, Kcal: 269

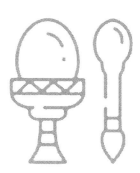

Ingredients:

- ◆ 4 slices of whole wheat, toasted
- ◆ 1 teaspoon white vinegar
- ◆ 4 eggs
- ◆ 6 tablespoons ricotta cheese
- ◆ 3 avocadoes, mashed
- ◆ 4 tablespoons harissa
- ◆ ¼ cup sliced green onions

Preparation:

1. Bring to boil a large skillet 1 ½ full of water, add a splash of white vinegar, and then break the eggs into the boiling water, being careful to space them out. Cover and turn off heat, leaving eggs in the water for 4 – 5 mins.

2. Toast the bread until slightly browned. Remove and set one side.

3. Add 1 ½ tbsp of ricotta, ¼ cup mashed avocado, and 1 tbsp of harissa to each slice of toast.

4. Gently remove poached eggs from water, draining any liquid, and place on top of assembled toast. Garnish with green onions and serve.

Six ingredient sausage potato pie

Time: 45 minutes | Serves 6 – 8

Net carbs: 66% (197g), Fat: 28% (18g), Protein: 55% (27.6g) , Kcal: 322

Ingredients:

- ♦ 350g ground sausage
- ♦ 6 to 8 eggs
- ♦ ½ cup milk
- ♦ 1½tsp herbs de Provence
- ♦ 450g raw, grated potatoes
- ♦ 1 cup grated cheese
- ♦ 2 cups kale, shredded
- ♦ Salt and pepper to taste

Preparation:

1. Pre-heat oven to 175°C (350°F). Use baking sheet to line a pie pan.

2. Cook and brown the sausage until crumbed, remove from heat and cool slightly.

3. Whisk the eggs, milk, herbes, salt and pepper. Add the hash browns, ⅔ cup cheese, kale, and cooked sausage and combine.

4. Pour into pie pan, topping with left over cheese and cover loosely with foil. Bake for 40mins/until potatoes are cooked.

5. Remove foil and bake at400/450°F (200/230°C) for 10 mins/until golden brown on top. Set aside for 10 mins until excess moisture is absorbed. Slice and serve.

Jelly 'n Peanut Butter Chia Pudding

Time: 1 hour 30 minutes | Serves 3
Net carbs: 19.1g, Fat: 13.3g, Protein: 6.1g , Fibre: 6g, Kcal: 211

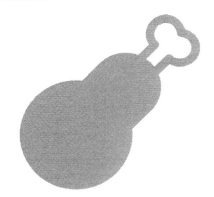

Ingredients:

COMPOTE

♦ 1 cup frozen/fresh wild blueberries

♦ 1tbsp orange juice

♦ 1tbsp chia seeds

CHIA PUDDING

♦ ½ cup light coconut milk

♦ 1 cup unsweetened plain almond milk

♦ 1 tsp vanilla

♦ 1 to 2 tbsp maple syrup to taste

♦ 3 tbsp salted peanut better

♦ ⅓ cup chia seeds

♦ Optional topping of fresh blueberries

Preparation:

1. Over medium heat, warm orange juice and blueberries using a small skillet/saucepan, until bubbling. Reduce to medium heat for 2 mins, stirring occasionally. Remove from heat. Stir in chia seeds.

2. Divide between 3 small serving dishes and refrigerator to set.

3. Blend on high to combine almond milk, coconut milk, vanilla, maple syrup and peanut butter. Taste and adjust to taste, adding maple syrup or peanut butter as required. Add chia seeds, pulsing carefully to ensure chia seeds remain whole. Set in fridge for 10 min to chill.

4. Remove both from the refrigerator. Stir chia pudding a stir and divide chia blend over the compote. Cover well and refrigerate for 1-2 hours/overnight/until chilled through.

5. To serve top with fresh blueberries and peanut butter.

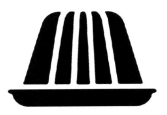

RECIPES FOR LUNCH

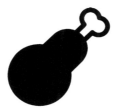

Grilled Chicken with Spinach and Melted Mozzarella

Time: 10 minutes | Serves 6

Net carbs: 3.5g, Fat: 6g, Protein: 31g, Fibre: 1.5g, Kcal: 195

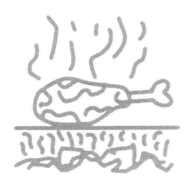

Ingredients:

♦ 680g (3 large) chicken breasts halved lengthwise

♦ 3 cloves crushed garlic

♦ 1 tsp olive oil

♦ 300g frozen spinach, drained

♦ 85g grated mozzarella

♦ ½ cup roasted red pepper, sliced in strips

♦ Olive oil spray

♦ Salt and pepper to taste

Preparation:

1. Pre-heat oven to 205°C (400°F). Lightly spray a grill/grill pan with oil. Add pepper and salt to taste to season chicken. Cook 2 to 3 mins/side.

2. Sauté oil and garlic in a heated skillet for 30 seconds over medium heat. Add spinach, salt and pepper, and cook for about 2-3 mins.

3. Topeach chicken breastwith spinach, mozzarella and roasted pepperson a baking sheet. Bake until melted (3 mins).

Eggocado

Time: 25 minutes | Serves 4
Net carbs: 9.2 (3.07%), Fat: 2.59g (12.95%), Protein: 3.86, Kcal: 185

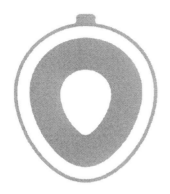

Ingredients:

♦ 1 extra large egg

♦ Juice of one lemon

♦ 2 avocadoes

♦ ¼ tsp paprika

♦ Pinch of freshly ground pepper

♦ ¼ tsp cayenne pepper

♦ ¼ tsp ground cumin

Preparation:

1. Pre-heat oven to 220˚C (425˚F).

2. Halve and de-pith avos and slice the rounded base to create a flat bottom on which to stand.

3. Whisk egg in measuringcup and season with salt and pepper.

4. Place the avocado halves on baking tray and pour egg mixture evenly into each half. Add a drizzle of lemon juice and sprinkle with salt, pepper, cumin, paprika, and dust with cayenne.

5. Bake for 18mins, or longer, to desired consistency.

Portabella Mini Pizzas

Time: 22 minutes | Serves 24 portions
Net carbs: 6g, Fat: 2g, Protein: 5g, Kcal: 67

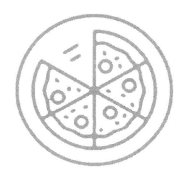

Ingredients:

- 150g chopped frozen spinach
- 1½ cup mozzarella cheese, shredded
- 1 tsp crushed dried basil
- ¼ tsp freshly ground coarse black pepper,
- 12 portobello mushrooms
- 2 diced medium tomatoes
- 2 tbsp margarine/butter, melted
- Pinch salt

Preparation:

1. Pre-heat oven to 175°C (350°F).

2. Once spinach is thawed and the liquid pressed out, chop it finely into a mixing bowl. Add cheese, basil and pepper.

3. Clean mushrooms and remove stems, place caps down on a lightly greased cookie sheet and brush with butter/margarine.

4. Drop 2 tablespoons of the spinach mixture into each cap and sprinkle with tomato and salt.

5. Bake for 12 mins/until heated through or place. Serve in quarters.

Venetian Shrimp and Scallops

Time: 20 minutes | Serves 4
Net carbs: 7, Fat: 17g (26%), Protein: 33g (66%), Kcal: 316

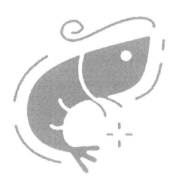

Ingredients:

- 450g sea scallop
- Coat pan with1tbspextra-virgin olive oil
- ¼ cup flour
- 2 cloves chopped garlic
- 1 large finely chopped shallot
- 2 tbsp butter
- 1 cup chicken brothand stock
- ½ tsp crushed red pepper flakes
- 140g-candiced tomatoes in juice
- 1cupdry white wine
- ¼ tsp saffron
- 450g deveined and peeled large shrimp
- basil leaves
- zest of 1 lemon
- Crusty, heated bread for mopping

Preparation:

1. Lightly coat sea scallops withflour seasoned with salt and pepper.

2. Coat preheated large skillet with oil and butter over medium high. Add scallops once the butter has melted into the oil. Brown scallops (2 mins each side) and remove from skillet.

3. Drizzle olive oil into the pan, and sauté garlic, shallots and red pepper flakes for 2 mins over reduced heat, stirring constantly.

4. Pour wine into a pan and reduce for a minute. Add stock, tomatoes and saffron threads and heat until bubbling before adding shrimp. Cook for 3 mins.

5. Add shrimp and scallops and cook for another 3 mins. Arrange shrimp and scallops on a warmed serving dish, garnish with lemon zest and basil. Serve with crusty sourdough bread and a salad.

Moroccan Meatballs

Time: 1 hr 30 minutes | Serves 6 – 8
Net carbs: 2, Fat: 21g (32 %), Protein: 17.14 g (34 %), Kcal: 273

Ingredients:

MEATBALLS:

♦ 900g ground lamb
♦ 2 tbsp shredded fresh parsley leaves
♦ 1 tbsp paprika
♦ 2 tsp ground cumin
♦ Salt and ground pepper

SAUCE:

♦ 1 tbsp coconut oil
♦ 2 med sized diced onions (2 cups)
♦ 2 tsp/2 minced garlic cloves
♦ 2 tsp paprika
♦ 2 tsp ground cumin
♦ 1 tsp salt
♦ ¼ tspground black pepper
♦ 2 medium diced tomatoes (2 cups)
♦ 1½ cups water
♦ ⅔ cup tomato paste
♦ 2 tbsp freshparsley leaves, shredded
♦ ¼ cup roasted pistachios, chopped

Preparation:

1. Combine parsley, paprika, cumin, salt and pepper. Crumble the lamb into the bowl and knead until combined. Moisten hands with water to roll a level tbsp of lamb into a ball between your palms. Set the meatballs aside once you have arranged them on a baking sheet.

2. Sauté onion in oil in a large pot/heavy skillet until soft (5 mins). Add garlic, paprika, cumin, salt, and pepper. Stir the mixture for half a minute until fragrant. Add tomato paste. Stir fry for 1 min. Add water, chopped tomatoes, and parsley and stir to combine. Bring to boil.

3. Gently place meatballs in skillet with sauce, cover, and simmer at reduced heat. Cook covered (40 mins). Remove lid and cook another 20 mins, until sauce is thickened.

4. To serve, sprinkle with chopped pistachios.

RECIPES FOR DINNER

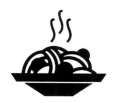

Cheese and Pepper (Cacio e Pepe) Spaghetti Squash

Time: 20 minutes | Serve 4

Net carbs: 3 % (8.3 g), Fibre: 7% (1.7g), Fat: 27% (17.3g), Protein: 22% (10.9g), Kcal: 228

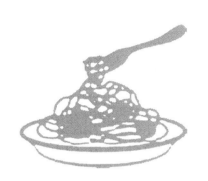

Ingredients:

- 1.8kg spaghetti squash
- 2 tbsp extra-virgin olive oil
- 1 cup Romano cheese, grated
- Pinch of salt
- Coarsely ground black pepper (to taste)

Preparation:

1. Cut squash in half, seed, and boil under tender (approx. 15 - 20 min).

2. In a bowl, set aside ½ cup cooking liquid. Drain and grate the squash and add to the bowl of liquid.

3. Toss squash in the reserved liquid. Dress with extra-virgin olive oil, cheese, salt, and lashings of black pepper. Serve.

One-pan cinnamon chipotle baked pork chops

Time: 30 minutes | Serve 4

Net carbs: 13.6g, Fibre: 3.5g, Fat: 7g, Protein: 25g, Kcal: 247

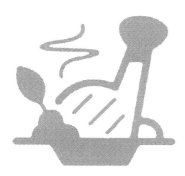

FOR THE PAN:

- 680g boneless pork chops/loin (4 pork chops)
- 2 to 3tbsp olive oil
- 2 large parsnips and 2 large carrots, sliced into ½ inch pieces
- Salt and pepper to season
- Garnishing: lemon slices, parsley, red chili pepper flakes

Ingredients:

CHIPOTLE RUB:

- 1 tbsp raw sugar
- 1 tsp ground chilli
- ½ tsp cinnamon
- ¼ tsp garlic powder
- ¼ tsp onion powder
- ¼ tsp smoked paprika
- Pinch dried oregano
- ½ tsp sea salt
- ¼ tsp ground black pepper

Preparation:

1. Combine chipotle in a small bowl, rub seasoning and set one side.

2. Preheat oven to 400°F(205°C). Arrange parsnips and carrots on baking sheet after tossing in olive oil and 2 tsp of cinnamon chipotle seasoning Roast for 15min.

3. Rub chops in cinnamon chipotle seasoning and sear in pan with 1 tbsp olive or avocado oil on medium high for 2-4mins. Turn once.

4. Remove chops from heat and arrange with vegetables on baking sheet. Replace in oven and roast/bake at400°F (205°C) for 6-8mins more.

5. Take the pan out of the oven. Garnish and serve.

Oven Roasted Cauliflower with Garlic, Olive Oil and Lemon Juice

Time: 35 minutes | Serves 4

Net carbs: 3% (8g), Fibre: 3g, Fat: 3g, Protein: 5g, Kcal: 89

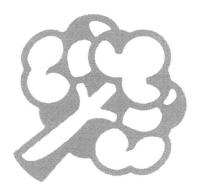

Ingredients:

- ¼ cup extra-virgin olive oil
- 5 or 6 cups cauliflower florets (1 medium cauliflower)
- 1tbsp sliced garlic
- ½ tsp ground black pepper
- ¼ tsp cayenne pepper
- 1 tbsp chopped fresh basil
- ½ teaspoon salt (optional)
- 2 tbsp lemon juice
- Salt and black pepper
- 2 tbsp grated parmesan cheese
- Garnishing: chopped chives

Preparation:

1. Pre-heat oven to 250°C (480°F).

2. Drizzle olive oil over cauliflower in large sauté/roasting pan. Add garlic, season with s & p, and drizzle lemon juice.

3. Roast the cauliflower florets for circa 10 to 15 minutes. Stir every three minutes to get evenly roasted florets. Remove from oven. Sprinkle with Parmesan and garnish with chopped chives. Serve while hot.

Spinach Souffle as easy as Pie

Time: 25 minutes | Serves 4

Net carbs: 20g, Fat: 17g, Protein: 14g, Fibre: 3g, Kcal: 274

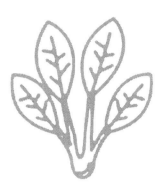

Ingredients:

♦ 1 egg

♦ ⅓ cup low fat milk

♦ ⅓ cup grated parmesan cheese

♦ 1tsp garlic, crushed

♦ 290g chopped spinach, thawed, & drained

♦ Salt and black pepper

Preparation:

1. Pre-heat oven to 170°C.

2. Whisk egg, milk, cheese, garlic, salt, and pepper together in a medium bowl. Fold in spinach and move to a small casserole dish.

3. Bake for 20 mins/until just set.

Spicy Garlic Shrimp in under 5 minutes

Time: 17 minutes | Serves 2

Net carbs: 2.8g, Fat: 17.7g (26%), Protein: 23.4g (66%), Kcal: 245.8

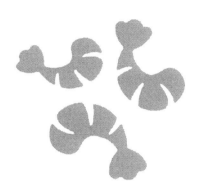

Ingredients:

- ♦ 12 jumbo shrimp & tails, peeled & deveined
- ♦ 2 crushed garlic cloves
- ♦ 2 tbsp olive oil
- ♦ ¼ tsp red pepper flakes
- ♦ 1 tsp steak seasoning of choice
- ♦ 1 tsp lemon zest
- ♦ 2 tsp lemon juice
- ♦ 1 tsp chopped fresh Italian parsley

Preparation:

1. Add olive oil, garlic, red pepper flakes, and shrimp to a large skillet heated over medium high heat.

2. Season with salt & pepper or grill seasoning. Cook shrimp for 3 mins/ or until just pink.

3. Toss with lemon juice, zest & chopped parsley and serve the shrimp on a serving platter without the garlic cloves.

RECIPES FOR DESSERTS

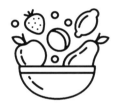

Low Carb trifle

Time: 20 minutes | Serves 4

Net carbs: 8g (9%), Fat: 34 g (86 %), Protein: 4g (5%), Fibre: 8g, Kcal: 368

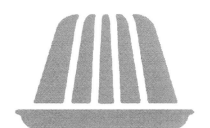

Ingredients:

- ◆ 1 ripe avocado
- ◆ ½ ripe banana
- ◆ 180ml coconut cream
- ◆ 1 tbsp lime juice and some of the zest
- ◆ 1 tbsp vanilla extract
- ◆ 75g fresh raspberries
- ◆ 60g pecans, preferably roasted

Preparation:

1. Place the avocado, banana, coconut cream, lime and half the vanilla in a bowl. Use an immersion blender or fork to mix together.

2. In a separate bowl, mix the remaining vanilla and berries.

3. Over medium heat, roast nuts in a dry pan, stirring frequently, until golden brown.

4. Alternate layers of the two mixtures in pretty glasses/bowls, top with nuts and serve.

Chocolate Mousse

Time: 20 minutes | Serves 4
Net carbs: 30g, Fat: 18g, Protein: 3g, Fibre: 3g, Kcal: 300

Ingredients:

FOR THE WHIPPED CREAM:

♦ ½ can coconut milk

♦ ¼ tsp almond or vanilla extract

FOR THE MOUSSE:

♦ 115g dark chocolate

♦ pinch salt

♦ 90 ml water

♦ Ice cubes from 1-2 trays

FOR THE GARNISH:

♦ coarse sea salt

Preparation:

1. Break chocolate in large chunks. Add the water and salt and place in a medium sauce pan on medium heat. Whisk until combined to a smooth, fluid, and shiny consistency. Turn off heat.

2. Place ice cubes and a cup of water in a large bowl. Add the hot chocolate to a smaller bowl and place it inside the large bowl. Whisk the mixture for 4 to 5 minutes to the ideal consistency.

3. Use a spoon to add the mousse to serving dishes. Serve immediately or refrigerate to serve later if serving with whipped cream.

4. For whipped cream, chill coconut milk beforehand. Spoon half into a chilled mixing bowl and add extract. Beatuntil the consistency of whipped cream(5 mins).

5. Top the refrigerated chocolate mousse with whipped cream. Add a dash of sea salt on top. Serve.

Banana Waffle

Time: 30 minutes | Serves 8

Net carbs: 4g (11%), Fat: 13g (75%), Protein: 5g (14%), Fibre: 1g, Kcal: 155

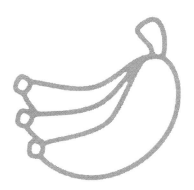

Ingredients:

- ½ ripe banana
- 2 eggs
- 2/5 cup almond flour
- 2/5 cup coconut milk
- ½ pinch salt
- ½ tbsp ground psyllium husk powder
- ½ tsp baking powder
- ¼ tsp vanilla extract
- ½ tsp ground cinnamon
- coconut oil or butter, for frying

Preparation:

1. Mix ingredients in a mixing bowl. Set aside for a while. Make in a waffle maker/pan fry with butter/coconut oil.

2. Place ice cubes and a cup of water in a large bowl. Positionaslightly smaller bowl inside the large bowl, scrape the hot chocolate sauce into the topbowland whisk (3-4 mins) untilthe desired consistency.

3. Spoon the mousse into serving dishes and refrigerate/serve immediately if not serving with whipped cream.

4. For whipped cream, chill coconut milk beforehand. Spoon half into a chilled mixing bowl and add extract. Beat until the consistency of whipped cream (5 mins).Dollop on top of the mousse, sprinkleapinch of coarse seasalton top. Serve.

   NOTES: Duplicate content. Check the recipe before it!

RECIPES FOR SNACKS

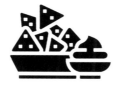

icy almond and seed mix

Time: 10 minutes | Serves 5

Carbs: 2g (6%), Fat: 15 g (81 %), Protein: 6g (13%), Fibre: 3g, Kcal: 166

Ingredients:

♦ 1 tbsp coconut oil or olive oil

♦ 125 ml almonds

♦ 40 ml (20 g) pumpkin seeds

♦ 40 ml (25 g) sunflower seeds

♦ ½ tbsp ground cumin or fennel seeds, crushed

♦ ½ tbsp chili paste

♦ ¼ tsp salt

Preparation:

1. Add chili to oil heated in a large frying pan, then add almonds and seeds, and stir thoroughly. Salt and sauté a while, being careful not to burn the almonds and seeds while developing the flavours of the spices.

2. Let cool down and then store in a glass jar.

Garlic Bread

Time: 20 minutes | Serves 20

Net carbs: 1g (3%), Fat: 9g (88%), Protein: 2g (9%), Fibre: 2g, Kcal: 92

Ingredients:

BREAD:

- ♦ 300ml/150g almond flour
- ♦ 40g ground psyllium husk powder
- ♦ 1 tsp sea salt
- ♦ 2 tsp/10gbaking powder
- ♦ 2 tsp cider vinegar/white wine vinegar
- ♦ 3 egg whites
- ♦ 225 ml boiling water

GARLIC BUTTER:

- ♦ 1 garlic clove, minced
- ♦ 110g butterat room temperature
- ♦ 2 tbsp finely chopped fresh parsley
- ♦ ½ tsp salt

Preparation:

1. Pre-heat oven to 175°C (350°F).

2. In a bowl, combine dry ingredients. Add vinegar, boiling water, and egg whites while whisking to a Play-Doh consistency using a hand mixer (30 seconds).

3. With moistened hands, form into 10 balls and shape into hot dog rolls. Arrange on baking sheet, allowing space for each to double in size. Bake on lower rack for 40-50 mins.

4. For garlic butter, combine all ingredients and refrigerate.

5. Remove the rolls from the oven. Let cool.

6. Remove garlic butter from fridge.

7. Halve the cooled rolls and spread with garlic butter, using serrated knife.

8. Turn heat up to 425°F (225°C) to bake garlic bread for 10 to 15 mins/ until golden brown.

RECIPES FOR SMOOTHIES

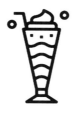

Peppermint Pattie Smoothie

Time: 5 minutes | Serves 1

Net carbs: 4g, Fat: 2g, Protein: 30g, Fibre: 3g, Kcal: 158

Ingredients:

♦ 1 cup unsweetened cashew milk

♦ ⅓ cup chocolate whey protein powder

♦ 1/4 tsp mint extract

♦ Handful fresh spinach

♦ 2 ice cubes

Preparation:

1. Blend ingredients until smooth using a blender. Serve in tall glass.

Choc Peanut Butter Smoothie

Time: 5 minutes | Serves 1

Net carbs: 6g, Fat: 24g, Protein: 33g, Fibre: 2g, Kcal: 604

Ingredients:

♦ 1 cup cold water

♦ ⅓ cup chocolate whey protein powder

♦ ⅓ cup heavy cream

♦ 2 ice cubes

♦ 2 tbsp peanut butter

Preparation:

1. Pre-heat the oven to 180°C (360°F).

2. Place all dry ingredients in a bowl and combine.

3. While whisking with a hand mixer, add vinegar, boiling water, and egg whites to the dry mixture. Whisk for about 30 seconds until reaching Play-Doh consistency.

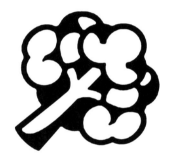

30 Day Meal Plan

"...and flour in all forms has to be eliminated forever. Bread isn't the staff of life in these times. Rather it is the staff of death."

— Blake F. Donaldson, Strong Medicine

Do you stand in front of your fridge before every meal, with no inspiration or idea what to prepare? Do you resort to stopping off on the way home for less than nutritious take-outs?

Do you battle to feed a family with different tastes and nutritional needs?

It is important with a meal plan to use it as guideline. It is not set in stone and you should adapt it according to your lifestyle and preferences. What is however important to minimise the carbohydrate intake and be cognisant of the nutritional value of the foods you eat.

With a properly compiled meal plan, you can solve all your problems with very little preparation.

This is an eating plan for 30 days, but low carb intake should ideally become a lifestyle to maintain health and fitness. Do not see this as a diet but rather a way of life going forward. You will learn to swop out meals and tweak the ideal meals to suit your days. Weekdays will probably be less of a problem than weekends but know that you can still eat out and have those drinks with friends on occasion.

DAY 1

Breakfast:

Classic Bacon and Egg

Serves 4| Duration 15min

Net carbs: 2 % (1 g), Fibre: 0 g, Fat: 75 % (22 g), Protein: 23 % (15 g), kcal: 272

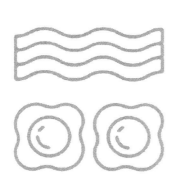

Ingredients:

- 8 eggs
- 150g bacon slices
- Fresh parsley and/or cherry tomatoes (optional)

Preparation:

1. Over medium high heat fry bacon until crispy. Set aside, leaving rendered fat in the pan.

2. Keeping the pan over medium heat, crack eggs into rendered fat, cooking eggs as desired (fried/scrambled/over easy/sunny side up)

3. Season to taste and serve with garnishing as desired

Lunch: Grilled Chicken with Spinach and Melted Mozzarella

Dinner: Cheese and Pepper (Cacio e Pepe) Spaghetti Squash

DAY 2

Breakfast: _One Minute Muffin_

Lunch:

Tuna salad with boiled eggs

Serves 2| Duration 15 mins

Net carbs: 2 % (6 g), Fibre: 5 g, Fat: 84 % (91 g), Protein: 14 % (33 g), kcal: 992

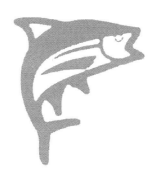

Ingredients:

♦   110 g celery stalks & 2 scallions,finely chopped

♦   150 g tuna in olive oil

♦   175 ml mayonnaise

♦   ½ lemon, zest and juice

♦   1 tsp Dijon mustard

♦   4 hardboiled eggs

♦   225 g Romaine lettuce

♦   110 g cherry tomatoes

♦   2 tbsp olive oil

♦   salt and pepper, fresh parsley

Preparation:

1. In a medium-sized bowl, combine celery, scallions, tuna, lemon, mayonnaise and mustard. Stir, season to taste and set one side.

2. Arrange tuna mix and hardboiled eggs on a layer of romaine lettuce. Add add tomatoes and drizzle with olive oil. Season to taste.

Lunch: One-pan cinnamon chipotle baked pork chops

DAY 3

Breakfast: Western-Style Breakfast Burritos

Lunch: Eggocado

Dinner:

Zucchini, tomato and cheese carpaccio

Serves 4 | Duration 7min

Net carbs: 12 % (10 g), Fibre: 4 g, Fat: 68 % (26g), Protein: 20 % (17 g), kcal: 348

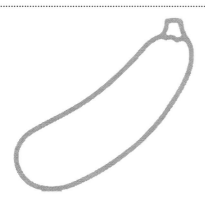

Ingredients:

- 4 tomatoes, chopped
- 2 zucchinis, sliced
- 4 tbsp capers, drained
- 200 g gouda cheese, in slices
- 4 tbsp (35 g) sesame seeds, toasted
- 4 tsp balsamic vinegar syrup
- 2 tbsp olive oil

Preparation:

1. Over medium heat, heat zucchini in olive oil until soft. Add tomatoes and season. Cook until the tomato is soft but not saucy (2 - 3 mins), add capers and simmer.

2. Cut cheese slices into rounds using a mould or cutter. Using a large ring mould, place vegetable mixture on plate and cover with a round of cheese. Top the cheese layer with balsamic syrup and sesame seeds.

DAY 4

Breakfast:

Egg butter with smoked salmon and avocado

Serves 4

Net carbs: 1% (5g), Fat: 83% (116g), Protein: 16% (50g), kcal: 1278

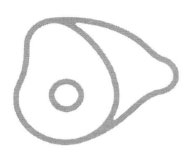

Ingredients:

- ♦ 8 hardboiled eggs, finely chopped
- ♦ 1 tsp sea salt
- ♦ ½ tsp ground black pepper
- ♦ 275 g butter, at room temperature
- ♦ 4 avocados
- ♦ 4 tbsp olive oil
- ♦ 2 tbspfresh parsley, chopped
- ♦ 225 g smoked salmon

Preparation:

1. Mix eggs and butter using a fork. Season to taste. Serve with a few slices of smoked salmon and diced avocado tossed in olive oil and finely chopped parsley.

Lunch: Portabella Mini Pizzas

Dinner: Oven Roasted Cauliflower with Garlic, Olive Oil and Lemon Juice

DAY 5

Breakfast: Poached Egg Harissa Avocado Toasts

Lunch:

Ham and cream cheese wraps

Net carbs: 27g, Fibre: 0 g, Fat: 9g, Protein: 17g, kcal: 250

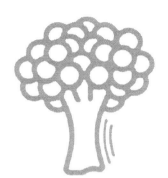

Ingredients:

- 4 x large Burrito Tortillas
- 120g spread cheese
- 1tbsp wholegrain mustard
- 2 tbsp chopped fresh chives
- 50g snow pea sprouts
- 100g shaved ham
- 1 carrot, peeled into ribbons

Preparation:

1. Incorporate the chives and mustard into the cream cheese.

2. On a clean surface, spread tortillas with cream cheese mixture. On the edge closest to you, position 2 slices ham, carrot and snow pea sprouts and gently roll. Secure with napkin/baking paper. Halve with serrated knife.

Lunch: Spinach Souffle as easy as Pie

DAY 6

Breakfast: Six ingredient sausage potato pie

Lunch: Moroccan Meatballs

Dinner:

Cauliflower risotto with roasted red peppers and burrata

Serves 4/15min

Net carbs: 3% (8g), Fat: 42% (27g), Protein: 23 % (16g), kcal: 310

Ingredients:

♦ 2 tbs butter & 1 tbs olive oil

♦ 450g riced cauliflower

♦ 115g roasted red peppers from a jar

♦ 120ml chicken broth or vegetable

♦ 1 tbs tomato paste

♦ ½ cup grated Parmesan

♦ 230g ball of burrata

Preparation:

1. Sauté cauliflower rice in olive oil and melted butter in large skillet for about 5mins, stirring frequently.

2. For puree, blend roasted red peppers in a blender until smooth.

3. Combine puree, broth & tomato paste with the cauliflower and cook to reduce, until cauliflower is tender. Add grated parmesan cheese and stir to melt. Season to taste.

4. Serve with ball of burrata sliced open in centre, in large serving bowl.

DAY 7

Breakfast:

Egg and Sausage Bake

Serves 4 | Duration 15min

Net carbs: 1 % (2 g), Fat: 123 % (80 g), Protein: 102% (51g), kcal: 948

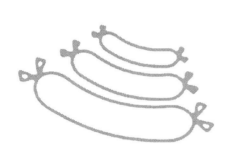

Ingredients:

- ♦ 2 cooked sausages chopped
- ♦ 2 eggs
- ♦ 1 tbs heavy cream
- ♦ ¼ cup grated cheese
- ♦ black pepper

Preparation:

1. Preheat oven to 375°F (190°C)

2. Add chopped sausage and cream to small baking dish. Crack the eggs over the sausages, careful to keep yolks whole.

3. Bake for 10 mins. Add cheese and bake for another 10 mins/until egg white is cooked.

Lunch: Grilled Chicken with Spinach and Melted Mozzarella

Dinner: Cheese and Pepper (Cacio e Pepe) Spaghetti Squash

DAY 8

Breakfast: Peanut Butter and Jelly Chia Pudding

Lunch:

Mummy Dogs

Net carbs: 2 % (1 g), Fibre: 0 g, Fat: 75 % (22 g), Protein: 23 % (15 g), kcal: 272

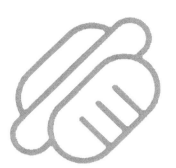

Ingredients:

♦ 1½ cups shredded mozzarella

♦ 2 tbsp cream cheese

♦ 1 egg beaten

♦ ¾ cup almond flour

♦ 6 beef frankfurters

♦ mustard/ketchup; seasoning

Preparation:

1. Preheat the oven to 380°F (200°C).

2. Microwave cream cheese and mozzarella for 1 min. Stir the mixture and cook for another half a minute until mozzarella melts completely. Add beaten egg, almond flour, salt and pepper. Mix well. Allow to cool before kneading for 1min.

3. Spread onto silicone. Cut into 12 long strips of dough. Wrap strip around frankfurter, then wrap another strip in the opposite direction in criss-cross pattern. Repeat with all frankfurters. Arrange on baking sheet. Bake (15-20mins) until dough is cooked. Serve warm, with mustard/ketchup.

Lunch: One-pan cinnamon chipotle baked pork chops

DAY 9

Breakfast: One Minute Muffin

Lunch: Eggcado

Dinner:

Cauliflower risotto with roasted red peppers and burrata

Serves 4/10min

Net carbs: 3% (8g), Fat: 42% (27g), Protein: 23 % (16g), kcal: 310

Ingredients:

- ♦ 2 tbs butter & 1 tbs olive oil
- ♦ 450g riced cauliflower
- ♦ 115g roasted red peppers from a jar
- ♦ 120ml chicken broth or vegetable stock
- ♦ 1 tbs tomato paste
- ♦ ½ cup grated Parmesan
- ♦ 230g ball of burrata

Preparation:

1. Sauté cauliflower rice in melted butter & olive oil in large skillet(5mins), stirring frequently.

2. For puree, blend roasted red peppers in a blender until smooth.

3. Combine puree, broth, and tomato paste with the cauliflower and cook to reduce, until cauliflower is tender. Add in grated Parmesan and stir until melted. Season to taste.

4. Serve with ball of burrata sliced open in centre, in large serving bowl.

DAY 10

Breakfast:

Greek Yogurt and Flax Pancakes with Berries

Net carbs: 3% (14g), Fibre: 0 g, Fat: 8% (11g), Protein: 16g, kcal: 228

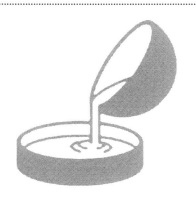

Ingredients:

- ♦ 1 cup blueberries
- ♦ 4 eggs, whisked
- ♦ 1 cup non-fat plain Greek yogurt
- ♦ 10 tbsp flax seed meal
- ♦ 2 tsp baking powder
- ♦ 4 tsp Stevia (or another sweetener)
- ♦ 1 tsp vanilla extract; 1 tsp cinnamon
- ♦ Salt

Preparation:

1. Simmer berries over medium heat in small pan (10 mins/until sauce consistency. Add sweetener if desired.
2. Mix eggs, yogurt, flax seed meal, baking powder, salt, sweetener, vanilla extract, & cinnamon. Set aside (5 mins) to thicken up.
3. Pour ¼ cup batter into non-stick skillet sprayed with cooking spray. Cook over medium high heat (3-4 min/side).

Lunch: Portabella Mini Pizzas

Dinner: Spicy Garlic Shrimp in under 5 minutes

DAY 11

Breakfast: <u>Western-Style Breakfast Burritos</u>
Lunch:

Creamy Southwest Chicken

Serves 4| Duration 25 mins

Net carbs: 3g, Fat: 13g, Protein: 15g, kcal: 191

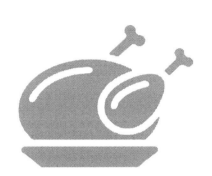

Ingredients:

- 2 boneless, skinless, medium chicken breasts
- 1 tbsp olive oil
- ¼ cup minced onion
- 2 cloves minced garlic
- 130g can green chilis, chopped
- ¼ cup cheddar, grated
- ¼ cup heavy cream

Preparation:

1. Place the oil in a medium skillet. Heat over low to medium heat. Sauté bite-sized chicken pieces seasoned to taste until brown on both sides. Add onions halfway through. Add garlic (cook 1min). Deglaze pan with water if necessary.

2. Add green chilis and cream. Simmer until sauce thickens and the chicken is cooked. Add a layer of grated cheese and serve when cheese is melted.

Lunch: <u>Spinach Souffle as easy as Pie</u>

DAY 12

Breakfast: <u>Poached Egg Harissa Avocado Toasts</u>
Lunch: <u>Venetian Shrimp and Scallops</u>
Dinner:

Tasty Zoodles

Serves 4/10min

Net carbs: 5% (15g), Fat: 29% (5.7g), Protein: 32 % (16g), kcal: 364

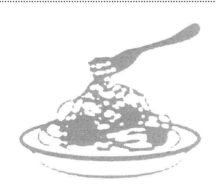

Ingredients:

♦ **1 medium zucchini spiralled with spiral maker (zoodles)**
♦ **1 cup fresh basil**
♦ **1 tbsp pesto**
♦ **Handful each cherry tomatoes & walnuts**
♦ **salt and pepper to taste**

Preparation:

1. Fry zoodles over medium heat in olive oil.

2. Halve cherry tomatoes and add to pan with walnuts. Toss. Cook for 7mins. Add pesto and toss again.

3. Serve with basil leaves as garnish or feta cheese if preferred.

DAY 13

Breakfast:

Sugar-free UP and Go

Serves 4 | Duration 15min

Net carbs: 8 % (25g), Fibre: 0 g, Fat: 77 % (50 g), Protein: 34 % (17 g), kcal: 581

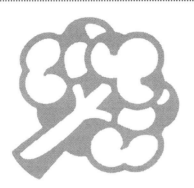

Ingredients:

- 500 ml milk -almond/coconut/full fat dairy
- 8 tbsp nut butter/almond butter
- 8 tbsp ground chia seeds
- 240 ml coconut cream
- 4 tsp vanilla
- 500 ml natural yoghurt unsweetened
- 8 tbsp granulated sweetener to taste

Preparation:

1. Blend all the ingredient in a blender/smoothie maker until thoroughly combined.

2. Serve immediately or store in a thermos for later.

Lunch: Moroccan meatballs

Dinner: Cheese and Pepper (Cacio e Pepe) Spaghetti Squash

DAY 14

Breakfast: <u>Six ingredient sausage potato pie</u>

Lunch:

Bacon and Pumpkin Soup

Serves 10 | Duration 4hrs 5 mins
Net carbs: 2% (5g), Protein: 2% (1g), kcal: 32

Ingredients:

- ◆ 1 bacon hock
- ◆ 900g pumpkin, diced
- ◆ boiling water

Preparation:

1. Cover the bacon hock and diced pumpkin with boiling water in the slow cooker. Cook on high for 3-4 hours or low for 6-10 hours/until meat starts coming away from the bone. Remove meat from bones. Return meat to cooker and discard bones.

2. Either serve as is or puree.

Lunch: <u>One-pan cinnamon chipotle baked pork chops</u>

DAY 15

Breakfast: Peanut Butter and Jelly Chia Pudding
Lunch: Grilled Chicken with Spinach and Melted Mozzarella
Dinner:

Simple Salmon

Serves 4/Duration 15min
Net carbs: 3.3g, Fat: 15.7g, Protein: 36.6g, kcal: 304

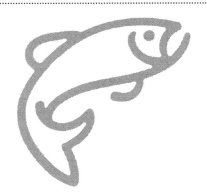

Ingredients:

- 1 tbsp garlic powder
- 1 tbsp dried basil
- ½ tsp salt
- 4 salmon (180g)
- 2tbsp butter
- 4 lemon wedges

Preparation:

1. Mix garlic powder, basil and salt to use as rub on the salmon fillets.

2. Cook salmon in melted butter in a skillet, over medium heat, until browned/flaky (5 mins/side). Serve with a lemon wedge.

DAY 16

Breakfast

Waffles

Serves 4 | Duration 20mins

Net carbs: 6g, Fibre: 3g, Fat: 22g, Protein: 14g, kcal: 264

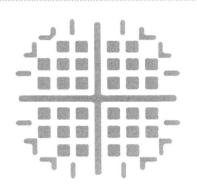

Ingredients:

♦ 4 large Eggs
♦ ½ cup Almond butter
♦ 1 tbsp sweetener
♦ ½ tsp baking powder

Preparation:

1. Blend all ingredients by hand or in a blender, until smooth.

2. Coat waffle maker lightly with oil/butter and preheat. Once the bubbles have settled in the batter, pour half evenly into waffle maker and close. Remove when done and repeat with remaining batter.

3. Serve according to taste.

Lunch: Eggocado

Dinner: Oven Roasted Cauliflower with Garlic, Olive Oil and Lemon Juice

DAY 17

Breakfast: <u>One Minute Muffin</u>

Lunch:

Beef Stroganoff

Serves 4 | 6 hrs 15 mins

Net carbs: 3 % (8 g), Fat: 29% (19 g), Protein: 58% (29 g), kcal: 317

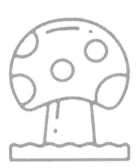

Ingredients:

- 1 brown onion sliced and quartered
- 2 cloves crushed garlic
- 2 slices streaky bacon, diced
- 500g beef stewing steak, cubed
- 1 tsp smoked paprika
- 3 tbsp tomato paste
- 250ml beef stock
- 250g mushrooms (quartered)

Preparation:

1. Place the ingredients in a slow cooker. Cook on low (6 to 8 hrs) or high (4 to 6 hrs).

2. Serve with sour cream.

Lunch: <u>Spinach Souffle as easy as Pie</u>

DAY 18

Breakfast: <u>Western-Style Breakfast Burritos</u>
Lunch: <u>Portabella Mini Pizzas</u>
Dinner:

Thai Salmon Fishcakes

Serves 2 | 18mins
Net carbs: 0% (1g), Fat: 18 % (12g), Protein: 72% (36g), kcal: 278

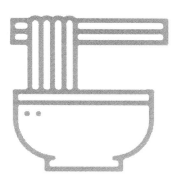

Ingredients:

- ♦ 2 salmon fillets, skin removed, 115g each
- ♦ 1 egg
- ♦ 2 tbs fresh cilantro roughly chopped
- ♦ 2 roughly chopped green onions
- ♦ ½ tsp red Thai curry paste
- ♦ Salt and black pepper

Preparation:

1. Using a food processor, mix the ingredients to a smooth consistency.

2. Divide mixture into 4, and spoon onto wax paper/baking parchment spread onto a plate. Cover with another layer of paper and plastic wrap. Refrigerate for one hour, minimum.

3. Fry fishcakes over medium heat in non-stick frying pan five mins per side.

DAY 19

Muesli

Serves 15 | min

Net carbs: 2% (6.1g), Fibre: 13% (3g), Fat: 27% (17.8g), Protein: 14% (6.9g), kcal: 200

Ingredients:

♦ 1 cup sunflower seeds
♦ 1 cup pumpkin seeds
♦ 1 cup sliced almonds
♦ 1 cup unsweetened flaked coconut
♦ ½ cup pecans
♦ 1tsp cinnamon
♦ ½ cup hemp hearts
♦ ½ tsp vanilla extract

Preparation:

1. Combine all ingredients well and lay on a rimmed baking pan. Bake at 350°F (180°C) for 7-8 mins. Leave to cool and store in a hermetic container.

Lunch: Venetian Shrimp and Scallops

Dinner: Cheese and Pepper (Cacio e Pepe) Spaghetti Squash (Page -)

DAY 20

Breakfast: Harissa Avocado Toasts with Poached Egg
Lunch:

Salmon, Avo & Arugula salad

Serves 4 | 7min

Net carbs: 4% (11g), Fibre: 28% (7g), Fat: 75% (49g), Protein: 50% (25g), kcal: 575

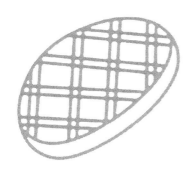

Ingredients:

- 85g arugula
- 225g smoked salmon fillet cooked
- 1 avocado
- Salad dressing
- ¼cup extra virgin olive oil
- 2tbs lemon juice
- 1 tsp white wine vinegar
- ½ tsp Dijon mustard
- black pepper

Preparation:

1. Mix all salad dressing ingredients together and set aside. Toss remaining ingredients in a bowl (salad bowl), drizzle with salad dressing and serve.

Dinner: One-pan cinnamon chipotle baked pork chops

DAY 21

Breakfast: Six ingredient sausage potato pie
Lunch: Eggocado
Dinner:

Spinach stuffed chicken

Serves 4 | 40min
Net carbs: 0% (0.8g), Fat: 42% (27g), Protein: 78% (39g), kcal: 271

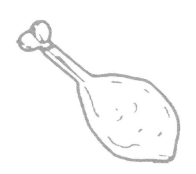

Ingredients:

♦ 4 chicken breast/fillets
♦ 4 tbsp cream cheese
♦ 2 slices cooked bacon, diced
♦ 1 handful spinach, cooked and drained

Preparation:

1. Slice each breast down the centre. Stuff with the spinach, cheese and bacon. Secure with toothpick.
2. Place breasts on oiled baking sheet and sprinkle with oil. Bake at 350˚F (180˚C) for 30 mins/until cooked in the centre.

DAY 22

Breakfast:

Spinach & Mushroom Omelette Muffins

makes 15 | 45mins
Net carbs: 2 % (5.06 g), Fat: 16 % (10.6g), Protein: 12% (6.17g), kcal: 148

Ingredients:

♦ ¼ cup butter

♦ 225g mushrooms sliced

♦ 150g fresh spinach

♦ 2 minced garlic cloves

♦ 2 tsp baking powder

♦ 2/3 cup coconut flour

♦ 7 large eggs

♦ ½ cup whipping cream

♦ 1 cup grated cheese

♦ Salt and pepper

Preparation:

1. Preheat oven to 350°F (180°C). Grease muffin pan.

2. Sauté mushrooms over medium heat in butter. Season with salt and pepper. Cook 5-7mins. Add garlic, cook 30 seconds. Add spinach and cook further minute until wilted. Set aside.

3. Add salt and pepper to coconut flour and baking powder.

4. Whisk together eggs, whipping cream and grated cheese. Whisk well and stir into mushroom/spinach mixture.

5. Spoon mix into muffin pan. Bake for 20 – 30 mins until puffy. Serve hot.

Lunch: Moroccan Meatballs

Dinner: Spicy Garlic Shrimp in under 5 minutes

DAY 23

Breakfast: <u>Peanut Butter and Jelly Chia Pudding</u>
Lunch:

Tuna Salad

Serves 4 | 15min
Net carbs: 3 % (9.4g), Fibre: 0 g, Fat: 14 % (9.3g), Protein: 32% (16g), kcal: 187

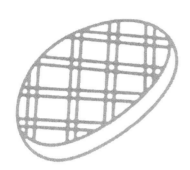

Ingredients:

♦ 2x 170g cans tuna in water, drained

♦ 2 tbs minced red onion

♦ 2 tbs minced celery

♦ 1 teaspoon minced parsley

♦ ⅓ cup prepared mayonnaise

♦ 1 tablespoon whole-grain mustard

♦ Freshly squeezed lemon juice (optional)

Preparation:

1. Shred tuna and toss with celery, onion, and parsley. Add mayonnaise, mustard and pepper to taste. Stir to combine and drizzle with lemon juice, if desired.

Dinner: <u>Spinach Souffle as easy as Pie</u>

DAY 24

Breakfast: <u>One Minute Muffin</u>

Lunch: <u>Portabella Mini Pizzas</u>

Dinner:

Poached Salmon
with Cucumber Noodles

Serves 2 | 15min

Net carbs: 2% (7g), Fibre 4% (1g), Fat: 66% (43g), Protein: 70% (35g), kcal: 556

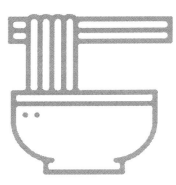

Ingredients:

- ♦ 1 tsp olive oil
- ♦ 2 salmon fillets
- ♦ ¼ cup unsalted butter
- ♦ 1 tbs olive oil
- ♦ 1 English cucumber
- ♦ ½ cup cherry tomatoes, halved
- ♦ 2 tsp lemon juice
- ♦ 4 to 6 leaves of fresh basil, finely chopped

Preparation:

1. In a pan, cook salmon in melted butter and olive oil for 10 to15 mins/ until cooked through), basting regularly.

2. Spiral the cucumber noodles using a julienne peeler or spiralizer. Place in a bowl and add olive oil, lemon juice, tomatoes, basil and black pepper to the "coodles". Mix well.

3. To serve, position salmon on a bed of cucumber noodles, sprinkling with black pepper.

DAY 25

Breakfast asparagus, with bacon and eggs

Serves 1/15min
Net carbs: 20.7g, Fat: 4g, Protein: 7.5g, kcal: 150

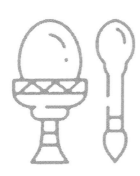

Ingredients:

♦ 2 slices bacon, diced

♦ 6 sprigs trimmed asparagus, discard woody bits

♦ 2 eggs

♦ ½ tablespoon chopped fresh chives

♦ ¼ teaspoon fine grain sea salt

♦ ⅛ teaspoon fresh ground pepper

Preparation:

1. Cook diced bacon in a cast iron skillet over medium heat (4 mins/until crispy). Place bacon on plate, leaving drippings in skillet.

2. Cook the asparagus in the hot pan until crisp & tender (5 mins). Crack 2 eggs over the asparagus and sprinkle with chives, salt and pepper. Sauté over medium-low heat until whites are set, and yolks are soft.

3. Add diced bacon and serve.

Lunch: Venetian Shrimp and Scallops

Dinner: Cheese and Pepper (Cacio e Pepe) Spaghetti Squash

DAY 26

Breakfast: <u>Western-Style Breakfast Burritos</u>

Lunch:

Creamy Southwest Chicken

Serves 4 | 25 mins

Net carbs: 3g, Fat: 13g, Protein: 15g, kcal: 191

Ingredients:

- ♦ 2 chicken breasts, without skin and bone
- ♦ 1 tbsp olive oil
- ♦ 1/4 cup onion (minced)
- ♦ 2 cloves garlic (minced)
- ♦ 130g can chopped green chilies
- ♦ ¼ cup heavy cream
- ♦ ¼ cup grated cheddar

Preparation:

1. In a large skillet, heat oil over medium heat. Sauté bite-sized chicken pieces seasoned to taste until brown on both sides. Add onions halfway through. Add garlic (cook 1min). Deglaze pan with water if necessary.

2. Add green chilies and cream. Simmer until sauce has thickened and chicken has cooked. Top with grated cheese. Serve once cheese is melted.

Dinner: <u>One-pan cinnamon chipotle baked pork chops</u>

DAY 27

Breakfast: Harissa Avocado Toasts with Poached Egg
Lunch: Moroccan Meatballs
Dinner:

Tangy Chicken Salad

Serve 1 | 15min

Net carbs: 20.6g, Fat: 10.5g, Protein: 27.1g, kcal: 286

Ingredients:

- 1 cup spring mix
- 1 cup romaine lettuce
- 1 tbsp chopped onion
- ½ cup mandarin oranges
- 1 tbsp dried cranberries
- 1 tsp. sunflower seed kernels
- 90g boneless skinless chicken breast
- 2 tbsp roasted red pepper dressing
- Salt, pepper, garlic powder to taste

Preparation:

1. Pat chicken dry and season on both sides. Grill/pan sear chicken until done. Set aside (3 mins), then slice against the grain.

2. Combined all ingredients and toss with dressing to serve.

DAY 28

Breakfast

Pancakes

Serves 2 | 10min

Net carbs: 1g, Fibre: 0 g, Fat: 37g, Protein: 38g, kcal: 500

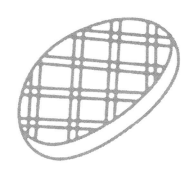

Ingredients:

♦ 2 scoops (50g) vanilla protein powder
♦ 2tsp baking powder
♦ 1 pinch salt
♦ 1 tbsp coconut flour
♦ 2 eggs
♦ ¼ tsp vanilla extract
♦ 4 tbsp unsalted butter (softened)
♦ 1 tbsp heavy cream

Preparation:

1. Combine dry ingredients and set aside. Combine eggs, vanilla, butter and cream until chunky. Fold in your preferred content now (bacon/ nuts/berries)

2. Ladle batter into a medium hot pan, coated with non-stick spray. Wait until bubbles pop before turning to cook other side (1 min). Serve.

Lunch: Grilled Chicken with Spinach and Melted Mozzarella

Dinner: Spicy Garlic Shrimp in under 5 minutes

DAY 29

Breakfast: Six ingredient sausage potato pie

Lunch:

Surprise me Salad

Serves 4/15 min

Net carbs: 2% (7g), Fat: 2% (1.5g), Protein: 8% (4g), kcal: 50

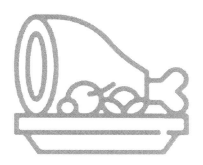

Ingredients:

- ◆ 1 handful fresh blueberries
- ◆ 1 cucumber, sliced
- ◆ 70g smoked salmon
- ◆ 1 tsp plain yoghurt
- ◆ 1 tsp soy sauce
- ◆ ½ tsp honey
- ◆ ½ tsp sesame seed oil

Preparation:

1. Stir together yoghurt, soy sauce, honey and oil to form dressing. Set aside.

2. Toss the berries, salmon slivers and cucumber slices into salad bowl. Drizzle with dressing and serve.

Lunch: One-pan cinnamon chipotle baked pork chops

DAY 30

Breakfast: Peanut Butter and Jelly Chia Pudding

Lunch: Eggocado

Dinner:

Steak and baked potato with salad

Serves 4

Net carbs: 51.8g, Fat: 7.1g, Protein: 70.1g, kcal: 700

Ingredients:

♦ 250g lean beef steak

♦ 4 x medium sized potatoes, baked

♦ 2 tbsp fat free sour cream

♦ Romaine lettuce, cherry tomatoes and cucumber slices

♦ Honey & Mustard salad dressing

Preparation:

1. Season the steak and grill to taste.

2. Top the baked potatoes with sour cream,

3. Toss the salad ingredients with salad dressing. Serve.

Disclaimer

The author's ideas and opinions contained in this publication serve to educate the reader in a helpful and informative manner. We accept the instructions may not suit every reader and we expect the recipes not to gel with everyone. The book is to be used responsibly and at your own risk. The provided information in no way guarantees correctness, completion, or quality. Always check with your medical practitioner should you be unsure whether to follow a low carb eating plan. Complete elimination of all misinformation or misprints is not possible. Human error is not a myth!

Imprint

Copyright © 2019
envdur.trade@gmail.com

Sarah Amber Patterson proxy of:
EnvDur Trading
Balat Mahallesi Rifat
Efendi Sokak, No: 19/1
34087 Istanbul
Turkey

Cover:
Design: Alima Media Turk
Image: Liliya Kandrashevich

42581285R00066

Printed in Poland
by Amazon Fulfillment
Poland Sp. z o.o., Wrocław